Natural Beauty Facials: Over 30 Homemade Facial Recipes You Can Make Tonight

Lisa Reinke

Cover photo licensed 9/5/20 with purchase # 192118462 by user ID 40193562 Lisa Reinke through:

Depositphotos Inc.

Address: 115 West 30th Street, Suite 1110B, New York, NY, 10001, United States

E-mail: support@depositphotos.com

Website: www.depositphotos.com Phone: +1-954-990-0075

Photo copyright held by MatoomMi (Janpen Chaiyadej).

Contact the author at: author@cheerful.com

ISBN: 9798684092565

Imprint: Independently published

CONTENTS

INTRODUCTION

Do you have a dressing table filled with products to help your beauty routine? Did they cost you a small fortune? Why not change your outlook and use the magical ingredients supplied by nature to make your own products? This book will show you how to turn some simple staple foodstuffs into refreshing, rejuvenating facial treatments. Learn what your skin type is and what products will be most effective for your routine. Turn your kitchen into a place that feeds both your body and your skin!

DETERMINE YOUR SKIN TYPE

Why You Should Determine Your Skin Type

Your skin is the largest organ in your body. It deals with exceptional stress and is subject to seasonality. Looking after it is just as important as maintaining a healthy heart, lungs, or liver. You need to choose the best cleaners and treatments to keep it in tip-top condition. If you use a cleanser that is designed for oily skin, you are telling your skin it has too much oil, while a cleanser that has excessive moisturizing properties can result in drier skin. You need to know exactly what your skin needs and what natural properties to apply to it. Everyone's skin is unique, but three common types will help you determine what products to use in your face masks. These skin types are commonly referred to as Dry, Oily, and Combination/Normal. We will address sensitive skin later in the book, but for now, we will concentrate on the three more common types. Be aware, however, that allergies can cause significant skin irritation. Before using large amounts of anything on your skin, try a small test patch on your inner wrist. I am allergic to cucumber, but I did not know that, and I put it directly on my face. Boy, did that hurt. Don't make my mistake.

How to Determine Your Skin Type

The Pared-Back Method

Clean your face thoroughly with warm water and a mild cleanser. Pat your skin dry with a clean cotton towel and let it dry naturally for 25 minutes. Now examine your skin for shiny areas or parts of the face that feels tight. Try your normal expressions like smiling and pursing your lips and check how your skin looks. If you have a noticeable shine on your forehead, nose, and cheeks, then you have oily skin. If your skin feels tight and flaky in these areas, you have dry skin. A shiny forehead and nose combined with dry cheeks and chin indicate a combination/normal skin type.

The Blotting Sheet Method

For a faster, more efficient way to determine your skin type, simply apply a sheet of blotting paper to relevant areas of your skin. If you have no evidence of moisture or oil on the sheet, then you have dry skin. Minimal oil on the forehead and nasal area indicate normal skin, and excessive oil means you have oily skin.

So, now you have determined your skin type, it is important to understand what this means for your cleansing routine. We will now examine what stand-alone products will help each skin type before we begin to combine them with other ingredients.

Dry Skin

These products will all help moisturize dry skin and should be included in natural face masks:
• Olive oil: This is one of the best natural cleansers as it will not strip your natural oils. You can just rub into your skin and then cover with a warm cloth until it cools. Remove the cloth and gently pat away the excess oil.
• Coconut oil: This is a great moisturizer for anything chapped. Dried lips, cracked skin, or dry hands will all benefit from applying coconut oil. Try using it as a makeup remover for a natural way to cleanse your face.
• Banana: Adding this fruit to your chosen oil will make it easier to apply and add extra moisture.
• Milk: Cleopatra certainly knew what she was doing when she bathed in milk! If your skin is feeling dry and irritated, take a carton of milk and pour some in a bowl. Use a clean washcloth for bathing the affected area for up to 5 minutes. The lactic acid in the milk should soothe the skin and prevent any further irritation.

Oily Skin

These natural products will help reduce the oil in your skin:
• Honey: You may not be aware of the term humectant, but it is an important term when treating oily skin. Honey is a natural humectant that draws moisture from the epidermis without replacing it. Using raw honey is a key benefit to oily skin that may be prone to breakouts.
• Oatmeal: When you have oatmeal for breakfast, it absorbs the milk and

forms a tasty dish. When used in skincare, it does the same thing with oil. Ground oatmeal mixed with warm water should be applied to the face with a gentle massaging motion. Repeat for up to 5 minutes and then rinse with warm water. Dry the face gently with a clean facecloth.

• Lemons: The acidic qualities in citrus fruits are helpful when treating oily skin. Combine with egg whites to make a gentle and easy to apply mask. Put the mask on your skin and leave to dry. Once the mask has dried completely, remove it with warm water and pat the skin gently dry.

Combination/Normal Skin

Combination/normal skin should be treated with both types of natural remedies, depending on the area being cleaned. Many different recipes are recommended for all three types of skin so let's explore the magical properties that could be sitting in your fridge, cupboard, or local store.

A Note on Essential Oils

Some of the masks in this book include essential oils. Essential oils should not be used directly on your skin or in the mask because they can cause irritation. You must dilute any essential oil you want to use in a carrier oil such as coconut oil, argan oil, jojoba oil, or almond oil. To do this, add 12 drops of essential oil to 1 ounce of carrier oil. Then you can safely add the mixture to your mask.

TOMATOES AND YOUR SKIN

If you open your refrigerator right now, what are the chances that you have tomatoes in there? Pretty high, right? So, do you make them into a tasty salad or fry them up to accompany your bacon for breakfast? Let's try something new and use them to improve your complexion and skin. Sounds radical, maybe.

Tomatoes are not the first thing we think of when it comes to face masks, but here are some of the amazing benefits they can provide your skin: 1) The natural acid in tomatoes helps you remove dull skin and promotes the growth of new cells. It also helps close pores and prevents the formation of blackheads and whiteheads. 2) Tomatoes contain a natural astringent that helps tighten the skin and reduce lines and wrinkles. 3) They contain a powerful antioxidant that helps prevent signs of aging. 4) When used as a cleansing agent, tomatoes leave the skin with a natural healthy glow. So, are you ready to embrace this natural fruit and make the most of its natural properties? Let's look at how to utilize these wonders of nature and treat different skin types.

Tomato Oily Skin Treatment

If you suffer from oily skin, try this simple mask to help you rejuvenate your skin and leave it soft, glowing, and free of acne.

Ingredients
• 1 ripe tomato
• 1 tbsp Fullers Earth (a clay that can be found in most good supermarkets, pharmacies, or through many online ecommerce websites)
• 1 tbsp mashed cucumber
• 1 tsp natural yogurt Make tomato puree in a blender or using a grater.

Combine with other ingredients until you have a manageable pulp. Apply to face and neck for 20 minutes before rinsing off. Repeat the procedure twice a week for optimum results.

Tomato Dry Skin Treatment

Try this versatile mask to restore vitamin E and essential fatty acids to your skin. This mask is especially effective for dry, mature skin types but can be used for all types of skin.

Ingredients
- 1 ripe tomato
- 2-inch piece of cucumber
- 2 tbsp almond flour

Place all ingredients in a blender and mix until smooth. If the liquid is too runny, add extra flour. Apply to face with upward strokes of the hand until your face is covered. Leave it to work for 10 minutes and then gently rinse your face. Pat dry. Use this mask twice a week for a glowing complexion with plumped up skin. It helps to restore the moisture you need to keep your skin healthy.

Tomato Combination/Normal Skin Treatment

If you have combination or normal skin, you may want to use the following face mask to aid smooth, flawless skin. It will help reduce puffiness and balance your natural pH.

Ingredients
- ½ cucumber
- 1 ripe tomato
- 1 tsp essential oil in a carrier oil (optional)

Blend or grate the cucumber and tomato to make a paste. Add a few drops of your chosen essential oil if required, and massage into your face. Use gentle strokes to spread the mixture onto your face and neck, then leave it for 15 minutes. Wash off gently and pat your skin dry. Try this rejuvenating mask every week to add a glow to your complexion and improve the appearance of your skin.

Tomato Face Mask

Ingredients
- 1 ripe tomato
- 1 tbsp manuka honey (a type of honey made in Australia or New Zealand by bees that pollinate the manuka bush)
- 1 tbsp olive oil
- 1 tbsp fresh lemon juice

Squeeze the tomato to release the juice and mash the remnants. Add the lemon and olive oil to the mixture and combine until smooth. Add the honey to form a paste and apply to the face and neck. Leave for 15 minutes to dry and then gently rinse off with cold water. Pat your skin dry with a clean towel.

Tomato Exfoliating Mask

Most people know that exfoliating is a great way to remove dead skin and stop the formation of blackheads and spots. Many products on the market will help you do this, but how can the humble tomato help? If you want to ditch the chemically treated products and go natural for exfoliation, try this simple, effective face mask:

Ingredients
- 1 ripe tomato
- 2 tbsp organic natural yogurt
- ½ tsp sugar

Cut the tomato into quarters. Sprinkle a little sugar on each section and top with a drop of yogurt. Rub your face and neck with the tomato until it covers the area you require. Wash off using cold water and then pat your skin dry.

The key to using tomatoes as part of your natural regime is to let your imagination loose. Don't just concentrate on your face; try them on other parts of your body. If you have excessively dry skin, try adding drops of essential oil like almond or argan oil for increased moisturization. Pampering your skin will help it glow. If you crave a natural way to make your complexion flawless, then reach for the tomatoes now! You will see a difference after just one use. If you want a quick, simple way to benefit from these super fruits, simply cut one in half and rub it on your face. Leave it for 15 minutes and then rinse off!

FRUIT-BASED FACE MASKS

Why do we eat fruit? Because it's tasty, good for us, or because it is packed with nutrients that make our skin glow? These reasons are also why we use natural chemical-free fruit masks to directly feed our skin. There is such a wide range of fruits to choose from, so indulge yourself and make some super healthy face masks immediately!

What Effect Do Different Fruits Have on The Skin?

We all know eating healthy is a great way to make our skin glow, but what about applying them topically. As we are discussing face masks, it is important to understand what different fruits do for our skin. This way, we can make simple recipes more effective by adding fruit that our specific skin need in the moment.

• Apples: These tasty fruits contain malic acid that helps the skin maintain a firm skin tone.
• Bananas: The potassium content helps skin moisturize while vitamins C and B5 help the skin maintain high levels of elasticity. They also help fade dark spots and circles beneath the eyes. Bananas help your skin look supple, fuller, and younger.
• Kiwi fruit: High vitamin C levels help the skin maintain collagen levels while vitamins in the flesh of the kiwi fruit are packed with high A, C, and E vitamins.
• Lemons: These citrus miracles help lighten the skin and clear pores. The citric acid brightens the complexion while replacing vitamin C.
• Papaya: This rich, fleshy fruit helps the skin fight free radicals that fight skin damage. It helps moisturize and replenish essential oils the skin needs.
• Watermelon: This fruit is one of the most hydrating ingredients possible.

It contains antioxidants and anti-aging contents that help circulation beneath the skin. The lycopene that gives the fruit it's red coloring also protects your skin from outside elements.

- Plums: These fruits are eaten to promote digestion, but when applied to the face, they release toxins from the skin.
- Pineapple: It is loaded with nutrients that include thiamin, potassium, and iron that all benefit skin health. The bromelain in pineapple is a natural exfoliant when used topically.
- Strawberries: Adding these awesome berries to your mask help you fight wrinkles and make skin smoother. They contain a salicylic acid that fights acne and penetrates deep into the pores. Strawberries also help give the skin a natural defense against UV damage.

Fruit Oily Skin Treatment

If you would like a mask that rids your skin of excess oil while hydrating and rejuvenating your epidermis, then look no further. Try these super zesty masks for a simple fix for oily skin. For oily skin, I suggest the sweet kiwi mask; the apple face mask; the lemon orange and pineapple face mask; and the pineapple, mango, and honey face mask.

Sweet Kiwi Mask

Ingredients
- 1 egg yolk
- 3 whole kiwis
- 1 tbsp olive oil

Use a clean cotton cloth to squeeze the juice from the 3 kiwi fruits and place the juice in a bowl. Beat the egg yolk into the juice and gently drizzle the olive oil into the mixture. Apply to your face and leave for 20 minutes. Use a warm damp washcloth to wipe the mask off.

Apple Face Mask

Ingredients
- 1 apple
- 1 egg yolk
- 1 tsp lemon essential oil in carrier oil

Mix well together and apply to the face for 10 minutes. Wash off with warm water.

Lemon Orange and Pineapple Face Mask

If you can resist the temptation of making a fruit salad, you will have a zesty, refreshing mask that will rid your skin of oil and leave it fresh and hydrated

Ingredients
- 3 slices of papaya
- 2 tbsp fresh orange pulp
- 6 pieces of fresh pineapple

Blend the mixture in a blender and spread it across your face with a gentle sweeping action. Let the mixture sit for 20 minutes before you remove it with warm water.

Pineapple, Mango, and Honey Face Mask

Ingredients
- 2 slices of papaya
- 2 slices fresh mango
- 1 tbsp raw or manuka honey

Warm the honey, so it becomes liquid while blending the fruit in a blender. Make it into a spreadable mash and apply it to the face for 10 minutes. Rinse off gently and then clean face with warm water.

Fruit Dry Skin Treatment

Fruit can be especially effective for dry, flaky skin that is prone to aging. Most fruits have moisturizing properties and can help plump the skin and make it appear more youthful. Try these amazing hydrating masks for glowing complexions in minutes. For dry skin, I recommend using the banana, papaya, and avocado mask; the pomegranate, honey, and banana mask; the raspberry, watermelon, and oatmeal mask; the peach face mask; and the strawberry face mask.

Banana, Papaya, and Avocado Mask

Great for exfoliating as it moisturizes, this mask is rich in oxidants and makes a colorful way to feed your face!

Ingredients
- 1 ripe banana

- 1 ripe avocado
- 3 slices of papaya

Use a potato masher to smash the fruits into a paste. Do not use a blender if you want to create a texture that will exfoliate as well as moisturize. Spread the paste vigorously over your skin with a massaging action to release dead skin cells. Keep the paste on for 10 minutes before washing off with warm water and then splashing cold water over the face. This helps close the pores and avoid impurities.

Pomegranate, Honey, and Banana Mask

Ingredients
- 1 whole pomegranate
- 1 tbsp raw or manuka honey
- 1 ripe banana

Deseed the pomegranate and place the seeds in a bowl. Mash the ripe banana with the seeds and add the honey. Gently use your fingertips to spread the mask evenly over your face and neck. Leave for 20 minutes and then use a warm facecloth to remove the mixture. Wash your face with warm water and let it breathe.

Raspberry, Watermelon, and Oatmeal Face Mask

Organic raspberries will help invigorate your skin and work with the oatmeal to help your skin glow with natural light.

Ingredients
- 1 cup of cooked oatmeal
- 2 slices of watermelon
- ½ cup of organic raspberries

Combine in a blender to form a smooth paste. Apply gently to the face and leave for 15 minutes. Wash off with warm water and then use cold water to close your pores.

Peach Face Mask

This mask is a good for anyone who wants younger-looking skin as peaches have anti-aging qualities.

Ingredients
- 2 ripe peaches
- 2 tbsp thick double cream, whipped
- 2 tsp almond essential oil

Mash the peaches and fold them into the whipped cream. Add the essential oil and apply it to your face. Use upward strokes to achieve a soothing effect on your skin. Leave to rest for 10 minutes and then rinse off with cold water.

Strawberry Mask

Strawberries are a rich source of folic acid as well as vitamin C. Try this simple mask to help raise your skin's metabolic rate as well as close dilated pores, only if you can resist eating it first, of course!

Ingredients
- 1 tbsp buttercream
- 6 mashed strawberries
- 1 tbsp blueberries

Combine the ingredients in a bowl without using the blender. Apply to your face and leave for 10 minutes. Rinse off with ice-cold water for a rejuvenating finish to your treatment.

Fruit is much more than part of your diet. Combine fruits to make amazing face masks, and your face will glow with a natural sheen.

HONEY-BASED FACE MASKS

Do you have a jar of honey in your kitchen? You probably use it for sweetening or for adding a burst of taste to your food. Honey has been around for millennia, and the first recorded beekeeping dates to 2400 BC and different cultures have been using it ever since. Honey has been used to dress wounds and treat ulcers for generations. It has effective properties that help the skin to heal and it also reduces pain. It has been used to treat burns and prevent infection for thousands of years. It also prevents scarring after wounds. Surely it makes sense to incorporate it into our facial cleansing regime. So, while you sit back and enjoy honey in your tea or use it to soothe a sore throat, you can also learn how to make all-natural skincare masks to give your complexion a healthy glow.

Honey Sensitive Skin Mask

If you have sensitive skin that can react badly when treated with some ingredients, you can make this healthy mask without worrying about adverse reactions.

Ingredients
• 1 tsp matcha powder (green tea leaves ground into a powder and available at health stores)
• 1 tbsp honey, preferably raw or manuka
• 1 tsp almond oil

Combining the green tea and honey means this mask will work anti-inflammatory magic on your skin. Combine the ingredients in a bowl and use a wooden spoon to mix. Once the mixture is smooth and even, apply it to the face and neck with gentle upwards strokes of the hand. Leave the mask to work on your free radicals for 15 minutes and then wash it off with clean, warm water. Pat, you face dry.

Honey Dry Skin Mask

If you have dry patches that are crying out for rehydration, try this mask to gently exfoliate while replacing essential moisture.

Ingredients
- 2 tbsp honey
- ½ avocado
- 2 tbsp ground hazelnuts
- 1 tsp essential oil in carrier oil

Combine the ingredients in a bowl and make a smooth paste. Apply to the face and neck with a gentle massaging action for 5 minutes. Leave the mixture on for a further 10 minutes before rinsing off with cold water.

Honey Oily Skin Mask

Clay masks are a fantastic way to control your oily skin, but it is unlikely you will have the ingredients to hand. It is worth the effort required to source the clay will make a huge difference to your skin, so visit your local health store or shop online for Moroccan red clay products. These ingredients will help you balance the natural oils in your skin and preventing breakouts.

Ingredients
- 1 tsp honey
- 1 tsp Moroccan red clay powder
- 1 tsp apple vinegar
- 1 tsp lemon juice

Mix the ingredients in a ceramic or glass bowl, as a metal bowl will react to the clay. Once the mixture forms a paste, apply it gently to the face and neck. After 10 minutes, wash your face with warm water. Once the mixture has been removed, splash cold water on your skin to close your pores.

Discolored Skin Face Mask

If you have dark spots or scars on your face, you can use honey to reduce the discoloration. This mask will also help disguise fine lines while exfoliating and promoting the growth of new cells.

Ingredients
- 1 tsp fresh lemon juice
- 1 tbsp honey
- 1 tbsp organic natural yogurt
- ½ tsp turmeric powder

Mix all the ingredients into a paste and spread a thin layer over the affected areas. Or you can cover your face completely with the paste. Leave the mixture to take effect for 20 minutes and then wash it off with warm water. This mask needs to be applied every week for around 12 to 15 treatments.

Nourishing Face Mask

If your skin looks dull and unhealthy, it may just need some nourishment. Just as the body needs food, so does your skin. Let's give it some much-needed love with this tasty treat straight from your kitchen!

Ingredients
- 2 tbsp cooked oatmeal
- 1 tbsp raw honey

Mix the two ingredients and apply to the face. Let the goodness sit for around 20 minutes and then use a warm washcloth to remove the mixture.

Radiant Face Mask

Do you wish you looked radiant? Do you want a glow that other people will comment on when they see you? Try this simple face mask to create that perfect glow!

Ingredients
- 1 tbsp raw or manuka honey
- 2 drops of lemon essential oil in carrier oil

Mix and apply to the face for 20 minutes then remove with warm water. Be careful to limit exposure to the sun for a day following the treatment as lemon juice can be oversensitive to sunlight and can harm your skin.

With all face masks, try a patch test, especially if you have sensitive skin and make sure you will not have a bad reaction. The honey you use should be as pure as possible, and raw honey is always the best option. Try mixing different essential oils to add your signature smell to a mask. Regular use of these natural products will improve your skin almost immediately.

VEGETABLE FACE MASKS

We all recognize the need to have our five a day for nutrition. A healthy mix of fresh fruit and vegetables to give our body the nutrients and vitamins it needs. So why shouldn't we do the same for our skin? Fruit is an obvious choice for refreshing, rejuvenating ways to feed your skin, but why not look at the vegetable options for a different way to get those important minerals and vitamins into your skin.

Dry and Aging Skin Treatment Options

For people with dry and/or aging skin problems, I recommend the kale face mask, the bell pepper face mask, and the cucumber face mask.

Kale Face Mask

If you feel your skin is looking dry and needs a boost, try this kale face mask to add moisture to your face.

Ingredients
- 4 large kale leaves
- 1 tsp oil
- 1 tbsp lemon juice

Add all the ingredients to a blender and mix until it forms a thick green paste. Apply to face and neck and leave for 20 minutes. Rinse off with warm water and then splash cold water on to close your pores.

Bell Pepper Face Mask

Another great alternative for dry skin is this colorful mask with bell peppers.

Ingredients
- 1 bell pepper
- 1 tsp whole milk
- 1 tbsp honey, raw or manuka whenever possible
- 1 tbsp of cooked oatmeal

Grate the pepper and add to a bowl. Add the other ingredients and mix into a smooth paste and apply to face and neck for 15 minutes. Wash off with warm water and rinse with cold water. If you require extra moisture, add a couple of drops of essential oil.

Cucumber Face Mask

If you feel your skin is looking tired and drawn, you should reach for a cucumber to make this refreshing mask. Make sure you have a suitable cloth to help the mask from drying too quickly.

Ingredients
- ½ cucumber grated
- 1 egg white
- 1 tsp lemon juice

Whisk the egg white until it forms a stiff peak and then fold in the cucumber and lemon juice. Apply to a clean face and neck area and cover with a damp cheesecloth or similar cotton fabric to help the mask stay moist. Leave on for up to 30 minutes and then rinse with cold water.

Oily Skin Vegetable Treatment Options

There are several options open to you if you have oily skin. I recommend using a zucchini treatment, cabbage mask, carrot mask, potato face mask, and beetroot face mask.

Zucchini Treatment

Zucchini is not just a tasty treat to add to your dinner plate. It has astringent properties that will help you remove excess oils and impurities from your skin. Here are two ways to use this humble vegetable to improve your complexion: Slice a small raw zucchini with a mandolin to create long thin pieces and put them directly on your face and neck. Wait 20 minutes and remove the vegetable slices. Wash your face with a mixture of clean water and cold whole milk to add moisture following your mask. Alternatively, you could grate the zucchini and add it to yogurt and oatmeal to create an excellent mask suitable for oily skin types.

Cabbage Mask

If you have both oily skin and acne scars or blemishes, you can benefit from the healing properties of cabbage.

Ingredients
- ¼ raw cabbage
- 2 tsp almond flour
- 1 tsp lemon juice

In a blender, mix the cabbage to create a wet pulp. Use a clean cotton cloth to squeeze the pulp to extract the cabbage juice. Thicken the juice with the almond flour and add the lemon juice. Apply the mask and leave for 15 minutes before washing it off with warm water.

Carrot Mask

Carrots are rich in vitamin C and can aid our diet, vision, and reduce the possibility of certain diseases. These qualities, combined with high levels of collagen, make it the perfect base for a DIY skin mask. This homemade mask is perfect for oily skin and will make your skin glow.

Ingredients
- 1 cup of grated carrot
- Corn starch to thicken
- 1 tbsp grated parsley

Mix and apply to clean skin. Wash off after 15 minutes with warm water and then splash the skin with cold water to close the pores. If you just feel like a boost, then all types of skin can benefit from the following masks. Make and apply to give your face and neck a tasty, colorful treat.

Potato Face Mask

Ingredients
- 1 medium potato
- 1 grated raw carrot
- 1 tbsp whole milk

Boil the potato with its skin on and leave to cool. Mash it thoroughly and add the milk and carrot. Once the mixture has cooled completely, apply it to your face and neck and leave for 10 minutes. Alternatively, you could grate raw potatoes and apply to the face and neck for a refreshing boost without the cooking!

Beetroot Face Mask

This mask is suitable for all skin types but should be made with yellow or white beetroot as the red variety will stain the skin.

Ingredients
- 2 tbsp grated yellow or white beetroot
- 1 tbsp Greek yogurt
- 1 tsp raw or manuka honey

Mix the ingredients and apply to face and leave for 30 minutes to work. Rinse with warm water and then splash with cold.

Once you have become a fan of vegetable face masks, you will recognize what works best for your skin. Try adding different elements to the masks above and create your own healthy creations.

YOGURT FACE MASKS

We all know how beneficial yogurt is to our diet. Natural full-fat varieties help balance our guts and aids in how we digest our food. Some cultures base their meals around natural dairy products, especially in the summer months. In Eastern Europe, a cold soup made with yogurt and cucumber makes a tasty alternative for breakfast. When we consider how yogurt affects our stomachs, it is just a short leap to making it part of our beauty regime. Even if you have an adverse reaction to eating yogurt, you can benefit from the effect it has on your skin. Yogurt is especially soothing if you are suffering from sunburn or other forms of tanning. It will calm your skin and remove the effects of damage caused by tanning. Here are some simple ways to make yogurt face masks that will work with all types of skin types.

Turmeric and Yogurt Face Mask

Turmeric is a plant originating in the Indian subcontinent that is known to have healing properties like antioxidants do, and it also has antibacterial elements. The soothing combination of yogurt and turmeric will help heal any skin-related problems while brightening your complexion as well.

Ingredients
- 1 tbsp Greek yogurt or organic plain yogurt
- 2 tsp organic turmeric available from most good supermarkets
- 1 tsp raw or manuka honey
- 2 tsp lemon juice or lemon essential oil

Mix roughly in a bowl and use the lemon juice to make a consistent paste. Apply 20 minutes before you plan to shower. Leave on your face until you are ready to shower and let the water remove the mixture as you wash.

Avocado, Blueberry, and Yogurt Face Mask

The creamy flesh of the avocado mixes with the yogurt to create a smooth paste that will help your skin to relax and glow. The mask will go deep into your pores and clear away any impurities. Blueberries add some vital antioxidants to the mask.

Ingredients
- 1 ripe avocado
- 10 ripe blueberries
- 1 tbsp organic yogurt

Add the ingredients to a blender and blend into a smooth paste. Apply the mask for 15 minutes then wash off with warm water. Splash cold water onto your face to close the pores and then pat dry with a clean cloth.

Gram Flour and Yogurt Exfoliating Face Mask

If your skin is feeling dry and flaky, it may help to exfoliate with this face mask. Gram flour, made from chickpeas, has been used for generations to clean the skin and make a perfect exfoliator. Suppose you require a more vigorous deep clean, add some Himalayan salt crystals to the mix. Gram flour also reduces the oxidation of DNA and proteins in the skin.

Ingredients
- 2 tbsp gram flour
- 2 tbsp organic yogurt
- 1 tsp Himalayan salt crystals (optional)

Mix the ingredients in a bowl and form a thick paste. Add more flour if required. Use your fingertips to apply the mixture using a massaging circular motion to apply the mask over your face and neck. Wait for the paste to dry before washing it off with lukewarm water. Splash cold water on your face to close the pores.

Oatmeal and Yogurt Face Mask

If you have issues like skin rashes, itchy skin, insect bites, or acne, you may need to try this mask. The oatmeal provides an effective emollient, while the yogurt leaves the skin smooth and fresh. The hypoallergic properties of the oatmeal will help your skin ward off any further attacks and will reduce blemishes.

Ingredients
- 1 tbsp ground oatmeal
- 1 tbsp Greek yogurt
- 1 tsp olive oil

In a bowl, combine the oatmeal and yogurt. Warm the olive oil on a spoon over a gaslight. Add to the mixture and stir until it forms a smooth paste. Apply to the face and neck with gentle pressure. Leve for 10 minutes and then wash with warm water.

Honey and Yogurt Face Mask

We already know honey is a key ingredient for dead skin removal but adding it to yogurt increases its effects considerably. The cinnamon and nutmeg will make your skin tingle and provide a natural source of oxygen.

Ingredients
- 1 tbsp raw honey
- 1 tbsp organic yogurt
- ½ tsp cinnamon
- ½ tsp nutmeg

Combine the ingredients in a bowl and apply it to your face with a clean brush. Leave for 10 minutes and then wash off with warm water. Pat your face dry with a clean towel.

As with most beauty treatments, natural face masks will have different results for everyone. Always perform a patch test before using any products on your face. Nature is an amazing supplier of products that can help you blossom. Remove those store-bought cosmetics and products and replace them with nature's bounty. Home remedies and homemade beauty products will not only be kind on your skin; they will also be beneficial for your pocket. Take advantage of the products in your fridge and cupboards and begin your natural journey to beauty!

CONCLUSION

Now you are ready to face the world with a complexion to envy! Treat your friends and family to the same experience and give your homemade face masks as gifts. Everyone loves a natural healthy glow, so share your knowledge and make the world a better place. Or you could just remain the envy of your friends and keep the secret to yourself! Good luck with your new beauty regime and happy blending.

GET MY NEXT BOOK FREE

If you want a free copy of my next book, please sign up to be on my VIP list by going to the website https://www.subscribepage.com/getafreebook

It would also help me out if you could leave a review for this book on Amazon.com. This is the link: https://www.amazon.com/review/create-review?asin=B08HHTWYMY

9 7 9 8 6 8 4 0 9 2 5 6 5